I0846367

Prevention Strategies
for
Kidney Infections

Prevention Strategies for Kidney Infections

Steps to Protect Your Kidneys

Victor Asher

Other Books by Victor Asher

Simple Exercise for Osteoporosis

Achieving & Maintaining a Healthy Life

The Inevitable Journey of Grief

Understanding the Quality & Benefits of a Revitalizing Sleep

A Step – By – Step Guide for Dads

Optimizing Life with Osteoarthritis

Unveiling The Hidden Benefits Of Walking And Hiking

Relationship's Hurricanes

Eating For Health

Cook well Eat well and live well

Exercise and Prostate Health

The Role of Nutrition in Osteomyelitis Healing and Prevention

The Enigmatic African Grey Parrot

Understanding & Taming the Fiery Nature of Anger

How to Achieve Financial Stability in Today's World

Coping with Adolescence

Alternative and Complementary Therapies for Rheumatoid
Arthritis

The Path to Success

Life Changing Quotes on Pages

Imaginative Tales to Dream Away

Beyond The Throne

60 Mind-loving Stories for Seniors

Dedication

This book is dedicated to God for His grace and wisdom, to my family, to my beautiful readers who will find this book relevant to them, and to everyone who has loved, supported, and encouraged me along the way. I would not be in the position I am in today without your unshakable faith in me. I dedicate this book to all my readers' especially those with kidney issues and desire to be healthy as this will sincerely be of importance to you all.

Table of Contents

Acknowledgement

I want to sincerely thank God for providing the means and insight that guided me during the writing of this book. I cannot forget my family members, whose encouragement and support have given me bravery and motivation throughout the process.

Thank you to my editor and publisher for their crucial advice and help in bringing this project to its successful conclusion. I would like to express my gratitude to everyone who so kindly contributed their time and knowledge to this project and added their wisdom. I want to express my gratitude to my friends as well, I appreciate all of your steadfast love and support throughout the journey.

I like to thank drsaurindalal.com, drmirdamadi.com and verywellhealth.com for those wonderful images, you all are wonderful.

Finally, I extend my thanks to each and every one of you for purchasing and reading my work. I am thankful it met your needs and added to your knowledge. I sincerely value each and every one of you and think you're all fantastic.

Introduction

Your kidneys are remarkable organs that silently perform crucial tasks to keep your body in balance. However, kidney infections can disrupt their harmonious functioning, leading to discomfort and potential complications. In the face of this threat, it becomes imperative to equip yourself with the knowledge and tools to protect your kidneys.

Welcome to "Prevention Strategies for Kidney Infections: Steps to Protect Your Kidneys," an empowering guide that unveils the secrets to maintaining optimal kidney health. Within these pages, you'll embark on a transformative journey of understanding, learning practical strategies, and embracing a proactive approach to safeguarding your kidneys against infections.

From the underlying causes and symptoms of kidney infections to the most effective prevention strategies, this comprehensive book leaves no stone unturned. You'll explore the power of good hygiene practices, the impact of a kidney-friendly diet, the role of hydration, and the importance of stress management in promoting kidney health.

But this book goes beyond mere prevention, it's a roadmap to empowerment. Armed with valuable insights and evidence-based recommendations, you'll discover how to make informed choices that align with your unique lifestyle and needs. With each turn of the page, you'll gain the confidence to take charge of your kidney health and create a solid defense against infections.

Written in a clear and accessible manner, "Prevention Strategies for Kidney Infections" is not just for those who have experienced kidney infections in the past. It's a call to action for everyone, urging you to prioritize your kidney health and prevent potential infections before they occur. By embracing the preventive measures outlined in this book, you'll be equipped to enjoy a life of vitality, free from the burden of kidney infections.

Get ready to unlock the transformative power of prevention. Let the pages of this book guide you towards a future where your kidneys thrive, and you revel in the knowledge that you hold the key to their protection. Are you ready to embark on this journey of empowerment? The time to safeguard your kidneys is now.

Chapter 1

The Kidneys

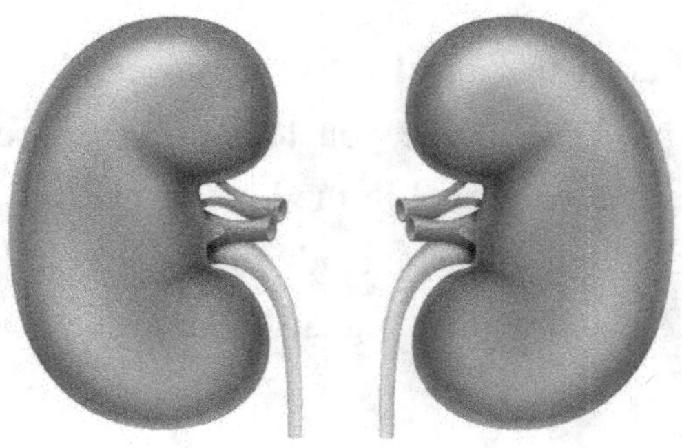

The kidneys are two organs that resemble beans and are each around the size of a fist. They are situated on either side of your spine, slightly below the ribs. Each kidney is encased in a hard, fibrous renal capsule that supports the delicate tissue within. Two additional layers of fat provide further defense on top of that, and over the kidneys are the adrenal glands.

The kidneys measure around 3 centimeters (cm) in thickness, 6 cm in width, and 12 cm in length. The typical weight of the kidneys in men is around 129 grams (g) for the right kidney and 137 g for the left. The average weight of these organs in females is 116 g for the left kidney and 108 g for the right kidney.

There are several pyramid-shaped lobes inside the kidneys. Each kidney has an inner renal medulla and an outer renal cortex. These portions are connected by nephrons. A filter called the glomerulus and a tubule are both parts of a nephron. Blood is filtered in the glomerulus after it passes through the kidneys' renal arteries and veins.

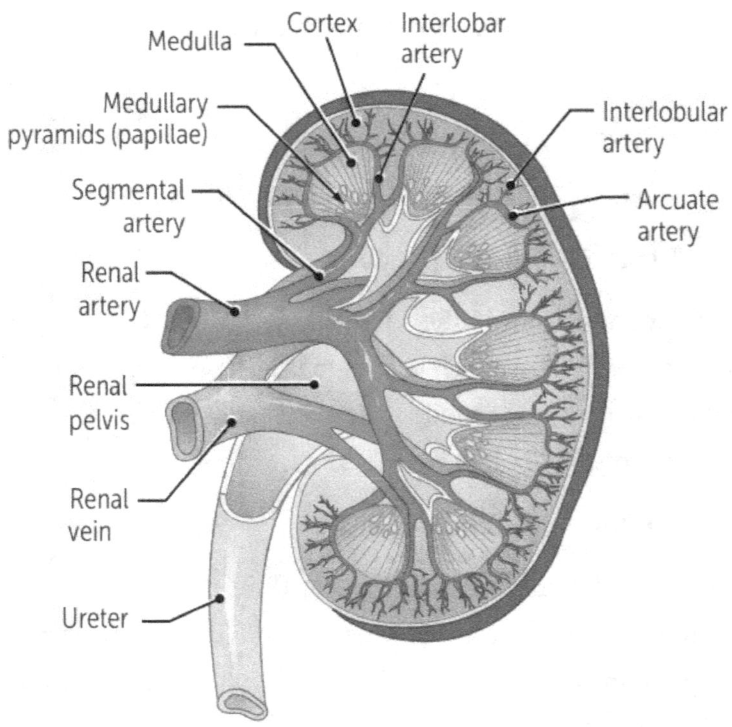

About a half cup of blood is filtered by healthy kidneys every minute, and this process removes wastes and surplus water to create urine and returns vital components to the circulation. The two skinny muscle tubes, or ureters, one on either side of the bladder, which carry urine from the kidneys to the bladder, are responsible for this process, as urine is kept in the bladder.

Despite being quite small, the kidneys get 20–25% of the heart's output.

Functions of the Kidneys

The kidneys are vital organs responsible for several essential functions in the body.

Here are the main functions of the kidneys:

1. Filtration of waste products

The primary function of the kidneys is to filter waste products, toxins, and excess substances, such as urea, creatinine, and ammonia, from the blood. These waste products are then eliminated from the body through urine.

2. Regulation of fluid balance

The kidneys help maintain the body's fluid balance by adjusting the volume and concentration of urine produced. They ensure that the body retains the necessary amount of water and electrolytes to keep blood pressure and bodily functions stable.

3. Blood pressure regulation

The kidneys play a key role in regulating blood pressure by controlling the amount of sodium and water reabsorbed into the bloodstream. They produce hormones like renin, which helps control blood vessel constriction and fluid balance.

4. Acid-base balance

The kidneys are involved in regulating the body's acid-base balance, which is crucial for maintaining proper pH levels in the blood. They can excrete excess acid or base through urine to keep the body's pH within a narrow range.

5. Red blood cell production

The kidneys produce a hormone called erythropoietin, which stimulates the bone marrow to produce red blood cells. Adequate red blood cell production is essential for carrying oxygen throughout the body and maintaining energy levels.

6. Vitamin D activation

Kidneys play a role in converting inactive vitamin D into its active form, calcitriol. Active vitamin D is crucial for calcium absorption in the intestines and maintaining strong bones.

7. Electrolyte balance

The kidneys help regulate the levels of essential electrolytes, such as sodium, potassium, calcium, and phosphorus, in the bloodstream. Proper electrolyte balance is essential for proper muscle function, nerve signaling, and overall cellular health.

8. Gluconeogenesis

In situations of prolonged fasting or starvation, the kidneys can generate glucose from non-carbohydrate sources (such as amino acids) through a process called gluconeogenesis. This helps provide a vital energy source for the body when carbohydrates are scarce.

9. Removal of drugs and foreign substances

The kidneys help eliminate drugs, medications, and foreign substances that are not needed or may be harmful to the body. They filter these substances from the blood and excrete them through urine.

In all, the kidneys are essential for maintaining internal homeostasis and overall health. Their functions extend beyond waste filtration to include fluid and electrolyte balance, blood pressure regulation, red blood cell production, and the activation of important hormones like vitamin D. By performing these critical functions, the kidneys help support the proper functioning of other organs and systems in the body.

Chapter 2

Understanding kidney infections: causes, risk factors, and complications.

A kidney infection, also known as pyelonephritis, is a painful and uncomfortable condition brought on when bacteria enter the urethra (the tube that expels urine from the body), ascends through the bladder, and get to the kidneys.

Kidney infections are typically caused by bacterial infections. When harmful bacteria enter the body and affect the kidneys, it results in a serious medical illness known as pyelonephritis. The kidneys are often affected once the infection has progressed from the bladder or urinary system.

The majority of the time, bacteria or viruses get inside the kidneys and cause infections. It has been hypothesized by researchers that the majority of kidney infections begin as bladder infections that then go up to affect one or both kidneys.

Typically, the upper urinary system is protected by the urinary tract's defenses from infections. For instance, when someone urinates, microorganisms are often flushed out before they enter the bladder. Urinary tract infections, however, can occur when the body's defense mechanisms falter thereby creating an avenue for microbes to advance and attack the kidneys if untreated.

The most common bacteria that can cause kidney infections include:

- *Escherichia coli* (E. coli): This bacterium is commonly found in the gastrointestinal tract and is the most common cause of urinary tract and kidney infections.

Other bacteria that can cause kidney infections, although less frequently, include:

- *Klebsiella pneumoniae*
- *Proteus mirabilis*
- *Enterococcus faecalis*
- *Pseudomonas aeruginosa*
- *Staphylococcus aureus*
- *Streptococcus species*

It's important to note that the specific bacteria causing a kidney infection can vary depending on factors such as the individual's age, gender, overall health, and any underlying conditions they may have. A healthcare professional can perform diagnostic tests, such as urine culture, to identify the specific bacteria causing the infection and determine the most appropriate treatment.

Signs and Symptoms

Kidney infections, also known as pyelonephritis, can cause a range of signs and symptoms. The common signs and symptoms of kidney infections include:

1. Fever

A high body temperature is a common symptom of a kidney infection. The fever may be moderate to high-grade and is often accompanied by chills.

2. Back or side Pain

Kidney infections typically cause pain in the lower back or sides. The pain may be dull and constant or sharp and intermittent. It is usually felt on one side of the back or abdomen.

3. Urinary symptoms

Kidney infections often present with urinary symptoms similar to urinary tract infections (UTIs).

These symptoms may include:

- Frequent urination
- Urgency to urinate
- Pain or burning sensation during urination
- Cloudy or foul-smelling urine
- Blood in the urine (hematuria)

4. Abdominal discomfort

Some individuals with kidney infections may experience abdominal discomfort, such as cramping, bloating, or a feeling of fullness.

5. Fatigue and weakness

Kidney infections can cause general fatigue and weakness, making you feel tired and lacking energy.

6. Nausea and vomiting

Some individuals may experience nausea, vomiting, or a decreased appetite as a result of a kidney infection.

7. Mental confusion (in severe cases)

In rare cases, severe kidney infections can lead to mental confusion or changes in consciousness. This is more common in older adults or individuals with weakened immune systems.

When a child under the age of two has a kidney infection, a high fever could be the only symptom. On the other hand, the typical symptoms of a kidney infection might not be apparent in persons over 65. Instead, elderly people may mostly face cognitive challenges, such as:

- Hallucinations
- Confusion
- Speech that is unclear or jumbled

It's important to note that the severity and combination of symptoms can vary from person to person. If you suspect you have a kidney infection or experience any of these symptoms, it is important to seek medical attention promptly. A healthcare professional can perform the necessary tests to diagnose a kidney infection and provide appropriate treatment to alleviate the infection and prevent complications.

Types of Kidney Infections

There are several types of kidney infections, each with its own characteristics and causes. Here are the main types of kidney infections:

1. Acute Pyelonephritis

This is the most common type of kidney infection and occurs when bacteria from a urinary tract infection (UTI) spread to the kidneys. Symptoms include fever, chills, back or abdominal pain, frequent urination, pain or burning during urination, cloudy or bloody urine, and fatigue.

While acute pyelonephritis is the main type of kidney infection, it can present in different forms based on the severity and location of the infection.

Some variations include:

- **Uncomplicated Acute Pyelonephritis**

This refers to a kidney infection that occurs in a healthy individual without any complicating factors. It can still cause significant symptoms and discomfort.

- **Complicated Acute Pyelonephritis**

This refers to a kidney infection that occurs in individuals with underlying health conditions or factors that increase the risk and severity of the infection. Complications may include urinary tract abnormalities, kidney stones, urinary tract obstructions, diabetes, pregnancy, weakened immune system, or recent urinary tract procedures.

- **Emphysematous Pyelonephritis**

This is a rare and severe form of acute pyelonephritis characterized by the presence of gas-producing bacteria in the kidney tissue. It can lead to kidney damage, abscess formation, and potentially life-threatening complications. Symptoms include severe pain in the abdomen or back, high fever, chills, nausea, vomiting, and altered mental status.

2. Chronic Pyelonephritis

This is a long-term kidney infection that causes persistent inflammation and scarring of the kidney tissue. It is often a result of recurrent or untreated urinary tract infections. Symptoms may be less pronounced compared to acute pyelonephritis and can include high blood pressure, frequent urination, pain or discomfort in the lower back or side, and recurring urinary tract infections.

3. Xanthogranulomatous Pyelonephritis

This is a rare and chronic kidney infection characterized by the presence of granulomas and fatty deposits in the kidney tissue. It typically occurs in individuals with a history of recurrent or untreated kidney infections. Symptoms may include fever, flank pain, weight loss, and malaise.

4. Renal Abscess

A renal abscess is a localized collection of pus within the kidney. It can occur as a complication of an untreated or inadequately treated kidney infection. Symptoms include fever, chills, back or abdominal pain, nausea, vomiting, and general malaise.

It is important to note that kidney infections can be serious and require medical attention. If you suspect you have a kidney infection or experience symptoms, it is recommended to seek prompt medical evaluation and treatment. A healthcare professional can diagnose the specific type of kidney infection and prescribe appropriate antibiotics or other treatments to alleviate the infection and prevent complications.

Risk Factors

Several factors can increase the risk of developing a kidney infection (pyelonephritis).

These risk factors include:

1. **Urinary tract abnormalities:** Structural abnormalities in the urinary system, such as vesicoureteral reflux (a condition where urine flows backward from the bladder to the kidneys), kidney stones, or urinary tract obstructions,

can make it easier for bacteria to reach and infect the kidneys.

2. **Urinary tract infections (UTIs):** UTIs, particularly recurrent or untreated infections, increase the risk of developing a kidney infection. Bacteria from the bladder can ascend to the kidneys and cause an infection.

3. **Gender:** Women are generally at a higher risk of kidney infections compared to men. This is because women have a shorter urethra, which makes it easier for bacteria to enter the urinary tract.

4. **Sexual activity:** Sexual intercourse can introduce bacteria into the urinary tract, increasing the risk of infection. One of such is anal sex and the risk is higher in women.

5. **Catheter use:** Having a urinary catheter, which is a tube inserted into the bladder, can introduce bacteria into the urinary tract and increase the risk of a kidney infection.

6. **Weakened immune system:** People with weakened immune systems, such as those with HIV/AIDS, undergoing chemotherapy, or taking immunosuppressant medications, are more susceptible to infections, including kidney infections.

7. **Diabetes:** High blood sugar levels in individuals with diabetes can impair the immune system's ability to fight off infections, including kidney infections.

8. **Pregnancy:** Pregnancy causes changes in the urinary system that can slow urine flow and increase the risk of urinary stasis, making pregnant women more prone to kidney infections.

9. **Age:** Elderly individuals may have weakened immune systems or underlying health conditions that increase the risk of kidney infections.

If you have any of these risk factors or suspect a kidney infection, it is important to seek medical attention for proper diagnosis and treatment.

Complications

Kidney infections (pyelonephritis) can lead to several complications, particularly if left untreated or not adequately managed.

Some of the potential complications include:

1. **Kidney damage:** A severe or prolonged kidney infection can cause damage to the kidneys. This damage may manifest as scarring, reduced kidney function, or the formation of abscesses (pus-filled pockets) within the kidneys.

2. **Sepsis:** Sepsis is a life-threatening condition characterized by a widespread infection throughout the body. If a kidney infection progresses and spreads to the bloodstream, it can lead to sepsis. Sepsis requires immediate medical attention and can cause organ failure or death if not treated promptly.

3. **Kidney abscess:** In some cases, bacteria can form abscesses within the kidneys. Abscesses are collections of pus that can cause pain, inflammation, and potentially rupture if not treated. They may require drainage or surgical intervention to resolve.

4. **Chronic kidney disease (CKD):** Repeated or severe kidney infections can contribute to the development of chronic kidney disease. Chronic kidney disease is a progressive condition in which the kidneys lose their ability to function properly over time. It may require long-term management or, in severe cases, dialysis or kidney transplantation.

5. **Hypertension (high blood pressure):** Kidney infections can disrupt the normal functioning of the kidneys, potentially leading to hypertension. High blood pressure can further damage the kidneys, creating a harmful cycle.

6. **Pregnancy complications:** Pregnant women with kidney infections are at an increased risk of complications, including preterm labor, low birth weight, and infection spreading to the fetus. Prompt treatment is crucial to minimize these risks.

It is essential to seek medical attention if you suspect a kidney infection to receive appropriate treatment and prevent the occurrence of complications. Timely diagnosis and management can help reduce the risk of long-term complications and promote a full recovery.

Chapter 3

Diagnosis of Kidney Infections

The diagnosis of a kidney infection typically involves a combination of medical history assessment, physical examination, and diagnostic tests.

Here are the common diagnostic methods used for diagnosing kidney infections:

1. Medical History and Physical Examination

Medical History and Physical Examination are essential components of the diagnostic process for various medical conditions, including kidney infections (pyelonephritis).

Here's a detailed explanation of each:

A. Medical History

During the medical history assessment, the healthcare provider will gather information about your symptoms, medical background, and relevant risk factors. They may ask questions such as:

- **Symptoms:** The healthcare provider will inquire about specific symptoms associated with kidney infections, including pain in the lower back or sides, fever, chills, urinary changes (frequency, urgency, or pain), nausea, or vomiting. Describing the onset, duration, and severity of symptoms can provide valuable insights.

- **Medical background:** They will ask about your medical history, including any previous kidney or urinary tract infections, history of kidney stones, structural abnormalities in the urinary tract, or other conditions that may increase the risk of kidney infections, such as diabetes or immune system disorders.

- **Risk factors:** The healthcare provider will explore potential risk factors that might contribute to kidney infections, such as recent urinary tract procedures, sexual activity, use of urinary catheters, or any other factors relevant to your situation.

B. Physical Examination

A physical examination allows the healthcare provider to evaluate your physical signs and assess specific areas associated with kidney infections. Here's what they might do:

- **Vital signs:** The provider will measure your blood pressure, heart rate, and temperature. Elevated temperature (fever) is a common sign of infection, including kidney infections.

- **Abdominal examination:** They will examine your abdomen, checking for tenderness, swelling, or pain. Special attention will be given to the areas around the kidneys, known as the flank region, which may exhibit tenderness or discomfort in the presence of a kidney infection.
- **Back examination:** The provider may perform a focused examination of your back, applying pressure or tapping (percussion) to identify any areas of tenderness or pain associated with the kidneys.

The combination of medical history and physical examination findings helps guide the healthcare provider in making a preliminary assessment and determining the need for further diagnostic tests, such as urine analysis, blood tests, or imaging studies.

It's crucial to provide accurate and detailed information during the medical history assessment and to cooperate during the physical examination to assist in reaching an accurate diagnosis and appropriate treatment plan. If you suspect a kidney infection or experience related symptoms, it is essential to seek medical attention for proper evaluation and care.

2. Urine Sample Analysis

Urine sample analysis is a key diagnostic tool used to evaluate kidney infections (pyelonephritis) and other urinary tract conditions.

Here is a more detailed explanation of the urine sample analysis process:

- **Collection of Urine Sample:** You will be asked to provide a urine sample in a sterile container. Proper hygiene measures should be followed to minimize contamination. In some cases, a midstream clean-catch technique may be recommended to ensure a representative sample.
- **Visual Examination:** The urine sample is visually assessed for color, clarity, and odor. Normal urine is typically pale yellow to amber in color, clear, and without a strong or foul odor.
- **Urinalysis:** This involves various tests to examine the physical, chemical, and microscopic properties of the urine. Key components analyzed include:
- **Specific Gravity:** This measures the concentration of the urine, indicating the kidney's ability to concentrate or dilute urine properly.
- **pH Level:** Determines the acidity or alkalinity of the urine.
- **Protein:** The presence of protein in the urine (proteinuria) may suggest kidney damage or inflammation.
- **Glucose:** The presence of glucose in the urine (glycosuria) may indicate high blood sugar levels, such as in uncontrolled diabetes.
- **Ketones:** The presence of ketones in the urine (ketonuria) may indicate the breakdown of fats as an energy source, often seen in uncontrolled diabetes or fasting states.

- **Blood Cells:** The presence of red blood cells (hematuria) or white blood cells (pyuria) in the urine may indicate inflammation or infection in the urinary tract.
- **Bacteria and Microorganisms:** Microscopic examination can detect the presence of bacteria, yeast, or other microorganisms that could indicate an infection.
- **Urine Culture:** If an infection is suspected, a urine culture may be performed. A small portion of the urine sample is cultured in a laboratory to identify the specific bacteria causing the infection. This helps determine the appropriate antibiotic treatment. The culture may also include a sensitivity test to determine which antibiotics are effective against the identified bacteria.

The results of the urine sample analysis, including the presence of abnormal levels of various components and the identification of bacteria or other microorganisms, aid in confirming the diagnosis of a kidney infection and guide appropriate treatment decisions.

3. Blood Tests

Blood tests are an important component of the diagnostic process for kidney infections (pyelonephritis). They help evaluate the overall health status, assess kidney function, and identify any signs of infection or inflammation.

Here are some blood tests commonly used in the diagnosis of kidney infections:

- **Complete Blood Count (CBC):** A CBC provides information about different types of blood cells. It can help identify signs of infection or inflammation, such as an elevated white blood cell count (leukocytosis). An increased number of white blood cells can indicate an active infection.

- **Blood Culture:** Blood cultures are performed to detect the presence of bacteria in the bloodstream. In severe cases of kidney infection or suspected sepsis, blood cultures may be taken to identify the causative bacteria and guide appropriate antibiotic treatment.

- **Kidney Function Tests:** Blood tests, such as serum creatinine and blood urea nitrogen (BUN), assess kidney function. Elevated levels of these substances in the blood may indicate impaired kidney function, suggesting possible kidney damage or dysfunction due to infection.

- **C - reactive protein (CRP):** CRP is a marker of inflammation. Elevated levels of CRP in the blood can indicate the presence of an infection or inflammation, including kidney infection.

- **Electrolyte Levels:** Blood tests can measure electrolyte levels, such as sodium, potassium, and chloride. Kidney infections can affect the balance of these electrolytes, and abnormalities may be observed in the blood works.

These blood tests provide valuable information to aid in the diagnosis and management of kidney infections. They help assess the severity of the infection, monitor the body's response to treatment, and evaluate any potential complications.

It's important to note that the specific blood tests ordered may vary depending on the individual's clinical presentation and the healthcare provider's judgment. If you suspect a kidney infection or have related symptoms, consult a healthcare professional who can order and interpret the appropriate blood tests for accurate diagnosis and treatment.

4. Imaging Tests

In some cases, imaging tests may be ordered to assess the structure and function of the kidneys. These tests can help identify any abnormalities, such as kidney stones or structural issues that may contribute to the infection.

Common imaging tests include:

- **Ultrasound:** This non-invasive imaging technique uses sound waves to create images of the kidneys and urinary tract.
- **CT scan:** A computed tomography (CT) scan provides detailed cross-sectional images of the kidneys, allowing for a more precise evaluation.
- **MRI:** Magnetic resonance imaging (MRI) may be used in certain cases to obtain detailed images of the kidneys and surrounding structures.

5. Additional Tests

In some situations, additional tests may be performed to determine the underlying cause of the kidney infection or assess for complications. These tests may include a renal scan, cystoscopy, or other specialized imaging or diagnostic procedures.

It's important to consult a healthcare professional for an accurate diagnosis and appropriate treatment. They will consider your symptoms, medical history, and the results of diagnostic tests to determine if you have a kidney infection and develop an effective treatment plan.

Chapter 4

Prevention of Kidney Infections

Prevention of kidney infections refers to the implementation of various measures and practices aimed at reducing the risk of developing pyelonephritis, a bacterial infection that affects the kidneys. Kidney infections can be painful and potentially serious if left untreated, causing complications and long-term damage to the kidneys. By adopting good hygiene habits, maintaining a healthy lifestyle, and being aware of potential risk factors, individuals can take proactive steps to minimize the chances of acquiring kidney infections.

These preventive measures encompass aspects such as proper hydration, hygiene practices, immune system support, safe sexual activity, prompt treatment of urinary tract infections, and avoiding irritants. While these strategies cannot guarantee complete prevention, they serve as valuable guidelines for promoting urinary tract health and reducing the likelihood of kidney infections. Regular communication with healthcare professionals and adherence to their advice can further enhance prevention efforts tailored to individual needs.

Preventing kidney infections, also known as pyelonephritis, involves adopting good hygiene practices and maintaining a healthy lifestyle.

Here are some essential steps to help prevent kidney infections:

1. Stay Hydrated

Drinking an adequate amount of water helps flush out bacteria and toxins from the urinary system. Aim for at least 8 glasses of water a day, or more if you engage in physical activity or live in a hot climate.

2. Practice Good Hygiene

Proper hygiene is crucial to prevent the spread of bacteria to the urinary tract. Always wipe from front to back after using the toilet to avoid transferring bacteria from the anal area to the urethra.

3. Urinate Regularly

Avoid holding in urine for prolonged periods, as this can allow bacteria to multiply in the urinary tract. Emptying your bladder regularly helps flush out any potential infection-causing bacteria.

4. Maintain a Healthy Immune System

A strong immune system plays a vital role in fighting off infections. Ensure you get enough sleep, exercise regularly, eat a balanced diet rich in fruits, vegetables, and whole grains, and manage stress effectively.

5. Practice Safe Sexual Activity

Engaging in safe sexual practices can help prevent sexually transmitted infections (STIs) that can lead to kidney infections. Use barrier methods, such as condoms, and communicate openly with your partner about sexual health.

6. Avoid Irritants

Certain substances can irritate the urinary system, making it more susceptible to infections. Minimize the consumption of caffeine, alcohol, and spicy foods, as these can irritate the bladder and urethra.

7. Urinary Catheter Care

If you require a urinary catheter, ensure it is properly inserted and regularly cleaned to minimize the risk of introducing bacteria into the urinary tract.

8. Promptly Treat Urinary Tract Infections (UTIs)

UTIs can progress to kidney infections if left untreated. If you experience symptoms such as frequent urination, burning sensation, or cloudy urine, seek medical attention promptly for appropriate diagnosis and treatment.

9. Avoid Chemical Exposures

Certain chemicals, such as harsh cleaning products and personal hygiene products, can irritate the urinary system. Opt for mild, fragrance-free alternatives to minimize the risk of irritation.

10. Regular Check-ups

Routine check-ups with your healthcare provider can help identify any underlying conditions that may increase your susceptibility to kidney infections. Follow their advice and take any prescribed medications as directed.

11. Regular Exercise

Exercise plays a supportive role in the management and recovery of kidney infections, but it does not directly treat or cure the infection itself.

Here's how exercise can be beneficial in the context of kidney infections:

- **Enhanced Immune Function:** Regular exercise has been shown to boost the immune system, which plays a crucial role in fighting off infections, including kidney infections. A strong immune system helps the body in combating the infection and promotes a quicker recovery.

- **Improved Circulation:** Exercise improves cardiovascular health and enhances blood circulation throughout the body, including the kidneys. Good blood flow helps in delivering oxygen and nutrients to the kidneys, supporting their function and facilitating the healing process.

- **Weight Management:** Maintaining a healthy weight is important for overall health, including kidney health. Obesity is a risk factor for kidney infections and other kidney-related complications. Regular exercise, along with a balanced diet, can help in managing weight, reducing the strain on the kidneys, and lowering the risk of complications.

- **Stress Reduction:** Kidney infections can be physically and emotionally stressful. Engaging in regular physical activity, such as aerobic exercises or yoga, can help reduce stress levels. Exercise promotes the release of endorphins, which are natural mood enhancers, leading to a sense of well-being and potentially alleviating the emotional burden associated with kidney infections.

- **Improved Urinary Function:** Exercise can stimulate urinary function and promote regular urination. This can help in flushing out bacteria and toxins from the urinary tract, potentially aiding in the recovery from kidney infections.

12. Eat a Balanced Diet

A balanced diet plays a significant role in the prevention of kidney infections in the following ways:

- **Nutrient Support:** A well-balanced diet provides essential nutrients that support overall health, including kidney health. Nutrients like vitamins, minerals, and antioxidants help strengthen the immune system, enabling the body to better defend against infections, including kidney infections.

- **Fluid and Urinary Health:** Adequate fluid intake is essential for maintaining proper urinary function and preventing urinary tract infections (UTIs) that can lead to kidney infections. A balanced diet includes foods with high water content, such as fruits and vegetables, which contribute to hydration. Additionally, consuming foods rich in fiber can help regulate bowel movements and prevent constipation, which can put pressure on the bladder and urinary system.

- **Blood Pressure and Blood Sugar Management:** A balanced diet that is low in sodium and refined sugars can help manage blood pressure and blood sugar levels. High blood pressure and uncontrolled diabetes are risk factors for kidney infections and kidney disease. By maintaining healthy levels, the risk of kidney-related complications can be reduced.

- **Protein Moderation:** Consuming an appropriate amount of protein is important for kidney health. However, excessive protein intake can strain the kidneys. A balanced diet ensures a moderate and balanced protein intake, supporting kidney function without overburdening them.

- **Sodium and Potassium Control:** Excessive sodium and potassium intake can negatively affect kidney health. A balanced diet focuses on limiting the consumption of processed foods and using less salt, helping to maintain optimal sodium and potassium levels in the body.

By adopting a balanced diet that includes a variety of nutrient-rich foods, adequate fluid intake, and moderation in protein, sodium, and potassium consumption, individuals can support their kidney health and reduce the risk of kidney infections. It's always recommended to consult with a healthcare professional or registered dietitian for personalized dietary advice, especially if you have specific medical conditions or concerns related to kidney health.

It's important to note that while exercise can offer several benefits in supporting overall health during a kidney infection, it's crucial to consult with a healthcare professional before starting or modifying an exercise routine. They can provide guidance based on individual circumstances, such as the severity of the infection, overall health condition, and any limitations or precautions that need to be considered. In some cases, exercise may need to be temporarily modified or restricted until the infection is fully resolved.

Remember, these preventive measures are generally beneficial, but they may not guarantee complete prevention of kidney infections. If you experience persistent symptoms or are at an increased risk, consult with a healthcare professional for personalized advice and guidance.

The role of cranberry juice and other natural remedies: separating myths from facts.

Cranberry juice and other natural remedies are often associated with preventing urinary tract infections (UTIs) and kidney infections. However, it is important to separate myths from facts regarding their effectiveness.

Here's an overview:

1. Cranberry Juice: Myth and Fact

Myth: Cranberry juice can cure or prevent UTIs. Some believe that the properties in cranberries prevent bacteria from adhering to the urinary tract, reducing the risk of infection.

Fact: While cranberry juice may have some benefits, scientific evidence supporting its effectiveness in preventing UTIs or kidney infections is limited. Some studies suggest a potential modest reduction in UTI recurrence, but more research is needed to confirm its efficacy. It is not a substitute for medical treatment or proper hygiene practices.

2. Natural Remedies: Myth and Fact

Myth: Various natural remedies, such as herbal supplements or essential oils, can prevent or treat kidney infections.

Fact: There is insufficient scientific evidence to support the effectiveness of most natural remedies in preventing or treating kidney infections. It is crucial to rely on medically proven treatments, such as antibiotics prescribed by a healthcare professional, to effectively treat kidney infections.

While natural remedies may have some anecdotal or historical use, it is important to approach them with caution and consult with a healthcare professional before using them for preventing or treating kidney infections. Proper hygiene practices, staying hydrated, and seeking medical attention for appropriate diagnosis and treatment are key in managing kidney infections effectively.

Chapter 5

Healthy Habits for Kidney Protection

The kidneys are critical to the body's ability to eliminate waste and toxins from the blood, maintain a healthy balance of fluid and electrolytes, and support numerous other key processes. Healthy Habits for Kidney Protection" refers to a collection of lifestyle activities and decisions that people can make to preserve their kidneys' optimum health and lower their risk of kidney-related illnesses and consequences.

You may safeguard your kidneys and enhance general health by practicing healthy practices.

Limiting alcohol consumption and quitting smoking: the impact on kidney health.

Limiting alcohol consumption and quitting smoking have significant positive impacts on kidney health as follows:

Limiting Alcohol Consumption:

- **Reduced Kidney Damage:** Excessive alcohol consumption can lead to various forms of kidney damage, including alcoholic hepatitis, alcoholic cirrhosis, and alcoholic nephropathy. Limiting alcohol intake helps reduce the risk of developing these conditions and minimizes the strain on the kidneys.

- **Blood Pressure Control:** Alcohol consumption can elevate blood pressure levels, increasing the risk of kidney damage and other cardiovascular complications. By limiting alcohol intake, individuals can better manage their blood pressure, reducing the burden on the kidneys.

- **Prevention of Dehydration:** Alcohol is a diuretic, meaning it increases urine production and can lead to dehydration if consumed excessively. Dehydration puts additional stress on the kidneys and impairs their ability to function properly. Limiting alcohol intake helps maintain adequate hydration, supporting kidney health.

Quitting Smoking:

- **Reduced Kidney Disease Risk:** Smoking is a significant risk factor for the development and progression of kidney disease. It can cause damage to blood vessels and reduce blood flow to the kidneys, leading to impaired kidney function. Quitting smoking lowers the risk of kidney disease and slows down its progression.

- **Lowered Blood Pressure:** Smoking raises blood pressure levels and damages blood vessels, including those in the kidneys. By quitting smoking, blood pressure can be better controlled, reducing the strain on the kidneys and promoting healthier kidney function.

- **Improved Treatment Outcomes:** If an individual with kidney disease continues to smoke, it can hinder the effectiveness of treatments and interventions aimed at managing the condition. Quitting smoking improves the chances of successful kidney disease management and slows down the decline of kidney function.

By limiting alcohol consumption and quitting smoking, individuals can significantly improve their kidney health and reduce the risk of kidney disease and related complications. It is important to seek professional support, such as counseling or support groups, for assistance in quitting smoking or reducing alcohol intake, if needed. Additionally, consulting with healthcare professionals can provide personalized guidance on lifestyle modifications and their impact on kidney health.

Managing chronic conditions: hypertension, diabetes, and other underlying diseases

Managing chronic conditions such as hypertension, diabetes, and other underlying diseases is crucial for preserving kidney health. Here's how effectively managing these conditions impacts the kidneys:

1. **Hypertension (High Blood Pressure)**
- **Kidney Function Preservation:** High blood pressure is one of the leading causes of kidney disease. Consistently

elevated blood pressure can damage the blood vessels in the kidneys, impairing their ability to filter waste and maintain proper fluid balance. By effectively managing hypertension through lifestyle modifications and prescribed medications, the risk of kidney damage can be significantly reduced.

- **Slowing Kidney Disease Progression:** For individuals already diagnosed with kidney disease, managing hypertension is essential to slow down the progression of kidney damage. Proper blood pressure control helps preserve kidney function and reduces the strain on the kidneys.

2. **Diabetes:**

- **Prevention of Diabetic Kidney Disease:** Diabetes is a major risk factor for developing kidney disease, known as diabetic nephropathy. Maintaining optimal blood sugar control is crucial in preventing or delaying the onset of diabetic kidney disease. This involves regular monitoring, adhering to a diabetic-friendly diet, and taking prescribed medications or insulin as directed, and engaging in regular physical activity.

- **Protecting Kidney Function:** For individuals with diabetic kidney disease, effective management of diabetes is necessary to slow down the progression of kidney damage. This includes regular monitoring of blood sugar levels, maintaining a healthy diet, adhering to prescribed medications, and managing other associated risk factors such as high blood pressure and cholesterol levels.

3. **Other Underlying Diseases:**

- **Comprehensive Management:** Many chronic conditions, such as autoimmune disorders or kidney-specific diseases, can impact kidney health. Effective management of these underlying diseases through appropriate medical treatments, lifestyle modifications, and regular medical follow-ups is crucial for preserving kidney function and preventing further complications.

- **Medication Management:** Some medications used to treat underlying conditions can have potential side effects on the kidneys. It is important to follow healthcare providers' recommendations regarding medication dosages, regular monitoring, and any necessary adjustments to minimize the risk of kidney damage.

By effectively managing chronic conditions like hypertension, diabetes, and other underlying diseases, individuals can significantly reduce the risk of kidney damage, slow down the progression of kidney disease, and preserve kidney function. Regular communication and collaboration with healthcare professionals are essential in developing personalized treatment plans and ensuring optimal management of these conditions.

Medication safety and kidney health: understanding potential side effects

Understanding potential side effects of medications is crucial for medication safety and kidney health. Here's an overview:

1. **Nonsteroidal Anti-Inflammatory Drugs (NSAIDs)**

- **Side Effects:** NSAIDs, such as ibuprofen and naproxen, can cause kidney damage or worsen existing kidney problems, especially when used in high doses or for prolonged periods. They can reduce blood flow to the kidneys and affect their ability to filter waste.

- **Precautions:** Individuals with kidney disease, hypertension, or heart failure should use NSAIDs cautiously or avoid them altogether. It's essential to follow the recommended dosage and duration of use and consult a healthcare professional if there are any concerns or preexisting kidney conditions.

2. **Antibiotics**

- **Side Effects:** Some antibiotics, such as aminoglycosides or certain cephalosporins, can be potentially toxic to the kidneys. They can cause acute kidney injury or increase the risk of kidney damage in individuals with preexisting kidney disease.

- **Precautions:** Healthcare professionals consider kidney function and adjust antibiotic dosages accordingly in individuals with impaired kidney function. It's important to inform healthcare providers about any preexisting kidney conditions or medications being taken.

3. ACE Inhibitors and ARBs

- **Side Effects:** Angiotensin-converting enzyme (ACE) inhibitors and angiotensin II receptor blockers (ARBs) are commonly prescribed for hypertension and certain kidney conditions. While they generally have kidney-protective effects, in some cases, they can cause a temporary decline in kidney function or increase potassium levels.

- **Precautions:** Regular monitoring of kidney function and potassium levels is essential for individuals taking ACE inhibitors or ARBs. It's important to follow healthcare providers' instructions regarding dosage and to report any symptoms or concerns promptly.

4. Diuretics

- **Side Effects:** Diuretics, such as loop diuretics or thiazide diuretics, can increase urine production and affect electrolyte balance, including potassium levels. They can occasionally lead to electrolyte imbalances or worsen kidney function in certain individuals.

- **Precautions:** Regular monitoring of kidney function, electrolytes, and blood pressure is crucial when taking diuretics. Adequate fluid and electrolyte intake should be maintained as prescribed by healthcare professionals.

5. **Contrast Agents**

- **Side Effects:** Contrast agents used for certain imaging procedures can potentially cause acute kidney injury, especially in individuals with preexisting kidney disease or risk factors such as diabetes or dehydration.

- **Precautions:** Healthcare professionals take precautions when using contrast agents in individuals with kidney impairment or at risk. Adequate hydration and monitoring of kidney function before and after the procedure are essential.

Understanding the potential side effects of medications on kidney health is important. It's crucial to communicate openly with healthcare professionals about any preexisting kidney conditions, medications being taken, or concerns about medication safety. Regular monitoring of kidney function, following prescribed dosages, and promptly reporting any changes or adverse effects are key for medication safety and maintaining kidney health.

Avoiding excessive use of over-the-counter pain relievers: risks and alternatives

To reduce the hazards connected with these medications and consider alternatives, it is essential to avoid abusing over-the-counter painkillers. Let's consider the follows:

1. **Risks of Excessive Use:**

- **Kidney Damage:** Regular or prolonged use of over-the-counter pain relievers like nonsteroidal anti-inflammatory drugs (NSAIDs) can increase the risk of kidney damage. These medications can reduce blood flow to the kidneys, impair their filtering function, and lead to kidney problems.

- **Gastrointestinal Issues:** NSAIDs, such as ibuprofen or naproxen, can also cause stomach ulcers, bleeding, and other gastrointestinal complications when used excessively or for extended periods.

- **Medication Overuse Headaches:** Frequent use of over-the-counter pain relievers can paradoxically lead to medication overuse headaches, where the headache becomes more frequent and severe due to the medication itself.

2. **Alternatives:**

- **Non-Medication Approaches:** Consider non-medication options for managing pain, such as applying heat or cold packs, practicing relaxation techniques, engaging in physical therapy or exercises, and utilizing topical creams or ointments.

- **Acetaminophen:** Acetaminophen (such as Tylenol) is an alternative pain reliever that is generally safer for the kidneys when used appropriately. However, it is important to follow the recommended dosage and precautions, especially if there are underlying liver conditions.

- **Lifestyle Modifications:** For chronic pain management, adopting healthy lifestyle habits can make a significant difference. This includes regular exercise, maintaining a healthy weight, managing stress, getting adequate sleep, and seeking alternative therapies like acupuncture or chiropractic care.
- **Consult a Healthcare Professional:** If pain persists or becomes chronic, it is important to consult with a healthcare professional. They can provide a comprehensive assessment, determine the underlying cause of the pain, and offer appropriate treatment options or referrals to specialists.

It is crucial to follow the recommended dosage and duration of use for over-the-counter pain relievers and consult with a healthcare professional if pain persists or if there are concerns about medication use. Remember, each individual's situation is unique, and personalized medical advice is essential for determining the most appropriate pain management strategy.

Regular check-ups and kidney function tests: early detection of potential issues

Regular check-ups and kidney function tests play a crucial role in the early detection of potential kidney issues. Here's why they are important:

1. Early Detection of Kidney Problems:

Regular check-ups with healthcare professionals provide an opportunity to assess overall health, including kidney function. Kidney diseases and conditions often progress silently without noticeable symptoms in the early stages. Regular monitoring through kidney function tests helps identify any abnormalities or changes in kidney function at an early stage, enabling prompt intervention and treatment.

2. Prevention and Management

Regular kidney function tests help identify risk factors and conditions that can potentially lead to kidney problems, such as high blood pressure, diabetes, or certain medications. By detecting these issues early, healthcare professionals can implement preventive measures, provide lifestyle recommendations, and manage underlying conditions to minimize the risk of kidney damage or slow down the progression of kidney disease.

3. Treatment Planning

Early detection of kidney problems allows healthcare professionals to develop an appropriate treatment plan tailored to an individual's needs. With timely intervention, treatment options can be explored, lifestyle modifications can be implemented, and medications can be prescribed to support kidney health and prevent further complications.

4. Monitoring Medication Effects

Some medications may have potential side effects on the kidneys. Regular kidney function tests help monitor the impact of medications on kidney health, ensuring that any necessary adjustments are made to the dosage or choice of medications to protect the kidneys.

5. Overall Health Assessment

Kidney function tests are part of routine check-ups and provide valuable insights into overall health status. They complement other health screenings, such as blood pressure measurement, blood glucose tests, and cholesterol checks. By monitoring kidney function, healthcare professionals gain a more comprehensive understanding of an individual's health, allowing for early detection of systemic issues or conditions that may affect kidney health.

By undergoing regular check-ups and kidney function tests, individuals can detect potential kidney issues early, facilitate prompt intervention, and enable effective management of kidney health. It is important to follow healthcare professionals' recommendations regarding the frequency of check-ups and screenings based on individual health status and risk factors.

Chapter 6

Kidney–Friendly Diet and Nutritional Tips

A kidney-friendly diet and nutritional tips are crucial for individuals with kidney disease or those looking to support their kidney health. This type of diet focuses on making dietary choices that promote optimal kidney function, reduce the risk of complications, and support overall well-being. By following a kidney-friendly diet and incorporating helpful nutritional tips, individuals can manage their condition effectively and improve their quality of life.

These dietary guidelines include considerations such as controlling sodium, potassium, and phosphorus intake, monitoring protein consumption, staying hydrated, and making nutrient-rich food choices. Working with healthcare professionals or registered dietitians can provide personalized guidance to tailor the kidney-friendly diet to individual needs.

Understanding the importance of a balanced diet for kidney health

A balanced diet plays a vital role in maintaining kidney health. They include:

1. Nutrient Support

A balanced diet provides essential nutrients, including vitamins, minerals, and antioxidants, that are necessary for optimal kidney function. These nutrients help support overall health and the proper functioning of the kidneys.

2. Blood Pressure Control

A balanced diet can help control high blood pressure, a leading cause of kidney disease. Consuming a diet rich in fruits, vegetables, whole grains, and low-fat dairy products, while limiting sodium, saturated fats, and cholesterol, can help maintain healthy blood pressure levels, reducing the strain on the kidneys.

3. Blood Sugar Management

For individuals with diabetes or prediabetes, managing blood sugar levels is crucial to prevent or delay the onset of kidney disease. A balanced diet that includes complex carbohydrates, fiber, and controlled amounts of carbohydrates can help regulate blood sugar levels and reduce the risk of kidney complications.

4. Weight Management

Maintaining a healthy weight is important for kidney health. Obesity is a risk factor for kidney disease. A balanced diet that focuses on portion control, moderation in calorie intake, and nutrient-dense foods can support weight management, reducing the risk of kidney-related complications.

5. Fluid and Electrolyte Balance

A balanced diet helps maintain proper fluid and electrolyte balance in the body. Consuming an appropriate amount of fluids, along with a diet rich in fruits and vegetables, supports hydration and electrolyte balance, which are essential for kidney function.

6. Reduction of Toxins and Waste Products

A balanced diet that limits the intake of processed foods, saturated fats, and artificial additives helps reduce the burden on the kidneys in processing and eliminating toxins and waste products from the body.

A balanced diet that includes a variety of fruits, vegetables, whole grains, lean proteins, and healthy fats provides the necessary nutrients to support kidney health. It is important to consult with healthcare professionals or registered dietitians for personalized dietary recommendations, especially if you have specific medical conditions or concerns related to kidney health. They can provide guidance on portion sizes, specific dietary restrictions, and individualized nutritional plans to promote kidney health.

Foods that promote kidney health: incorporating fruits, vegetables, and whole grains

Incorporating fruits, vegetables, and whole grains into your diet can promote kidney health. Here's how these foods contribute:

1. **Fruits**
*   **Antioxidants and Phytochemicals**

Fruits are rich in antioxidants and phytochemicals, which help protect against cell damage and inflammation. This can be beneficial for kidney health as inflammation and oxidative stress can contribute to kidney damage.

*   **Hydration Support**

Many fruits have high water content, contributing to proper hydration. Staying well-hydrated is essential for maintaining optimal kidney function and preventing complications like kidney stones.

2. **Vegetables**
*   **Nutrient-Rich**

Vegetables are packed with essential vitamins, minerals, and fiber. They provide important nutrients that support overall health, including kidney function.

*   **Lower Sodium Content**

Many vegetables are naturally low in sodium, which is beneficial for managing blood pressure and reducing the strain on the kidneys.

3. **Whole Grains**
- **Fiber Content**

Whole grains are an excellent source of dietary fiber, which helps regulate digestion, promote bowel regularity, and prevent constipation. This indirectly supports kidney health by reducing the risk of urinary tract infections.

- **Lower Glycemic Index**

Whole grains have a lower glycemic index compared to refined grains, meaning they have a smaller impact on blood sugar levels. This is important for individuals with diabetes or prediabetes, as uncontrolled blood sugar levels can lead to kidney damage.

It's important to note that individual dietary needs may vary based on specific health conditions and medical advice. Consulting with a healthcare professional or registered dietitian can provide personalized guidance on incorporating fruits, vegetables, and whole grains into your diet while considering any specific dietary restrictions or recommendations.

Limiting sodium, processed foods, and added sugars: their impact on kidney function

Limiting sodium, processed foods, and added sugars can have a positive impact on kidney function such as follows:

1. **Sodium**
- **Blood Pressure Control**

Excessive sodium intake can contribute to high blood pressure, a leading cause of kidney disease. By reducing sodium consumption, blood pressure can be better controlled, reducing the strain on the kidneys and minimizing the risk of kidney damage.

- Fluid Balance

Sodium plays a role in regulating fluid balance in the body. Consuming too much sodium can disrupt this balance and lead to fluid retention, putting additional stress on the kidneys. Limiting sodium helps maintain proper fluid balance and supports optimal kidney function.

2. Processed Foods

- **High Sodium Content**

Processed foods, such as canned soups, processed meats, and packaged snacks, are often high in sodium. Consuming these foods regularly can contribute to elevated sodium levels and increase the risk of high blood pressure and kidney damage.

- **Lack of Nutrients**

Processed foods are typically low in essential nutrients and fiber, which are important for overall health, including kidney function. Choosing fresh, whole foods instead of processed options ensures a higher intake of beneficial nutrients.

3. Added Sugars

- **Diabetes Prevention**

Excessive consumption of added sugars, particularly in sugary beverages and processed snacks, can contribute to obesity and the development of type 2 diabetes. Uncontrolled diabetes is a major risk factor for kidney disease.

- **Blood Sugar Control**

Managing blood sugar levels is crucial for individuals with diabetes or prediabetes to prevent kidney damage. By reducing added sugars, blood sugar levels can be better regulated, reducing the risk of kidney complications.

By limiting sodium, processed foods, and added sugars, individuals can support kidney health by managing blood pressure, promoting proper fluid balance, reducing the risk of diabetes, and ensuring a nutrient-rich diet. Opting for fresh, whole foods and preparing meals at home using natural ingredients can significantly contribute to a healthier diet and kidney function. It's important to consult with a healthcare professional or registered dietitian for personalized guidance on dietary modifications based on individual health conditions and needs.

The role of specific nutrients: potassium, phosphorus, and protein

Specific nutrients like potassium, phosphorus, and protein play important roles in kidney health. Here's an overview of their significance:

1. Potassium
- **Maintaining Electrolyte Balance**

Potassium is an essential electrolyte that helps maintain proper fluid balance and supports nerve and muscle function, including the heart. However, individuals with kidney disease may experience difficulty in regulating potassium levels, leading to imbalances.

- **Dietary Considerations**

In advanced kidney disease, high potassium levels (hyperkalemia) can be problematic. In such cases, healthcare professionals may recommend limiting potassium-rich foods such as bananas, oranges, potatoes, tomatoes, and leafy greens. However, for individuals with normal kidney function, consuming potassium-rich foods as part of a balanced diet is generally beneficial.

2. Phosphorus
- **Bone Health and Mineral Balance**

Phosphorus plays a crucial role in bone health and the formation of ATP (energy molecule) in the body.

However, individuals with kidney disease often experience difficulty in effectively excreting excess phosphorus, leading to elevated levels.

- **Dietary Considerations**

To manage phosphorus levels, individuals with kidney disease may need to limit high-phosphorus foods such as dairy products, processed meats, carbonated beverages, and certain nuts and seeds. Controlling phosphorus intake through diet and, if necessary, phosphate binders prescribed by healthcare professionals can help prevent complications associated with high phosphorus levels.

3. **Protein**
- **Building Blocks and Waste Production**

Protein is essential for tissue repair, immune function, and overall health. However, excessive protein intake can strain the kidneys due to increased waste products generated during protein metabolism.

- **Dietary Considerations**

Individuals with kidney disease may be advised to monitor and adjust their protein intake based on their kidney function and the stage of the disease. Healthcare professionals or registered dietitians can provide personalized recommendations regarding the optimal amount and sources of protein to balance nutritional needs while minimizing strain on the kidneys.

It's important to note that the specific dietary considerations for potassium, phosphorus, and protein can vary based on an individual's kidney function, stage of kidney disease, and overall health status. Regular monitoring and consultation with healthcare professionals or registered dietitians are crucial for personalized dietary guidance and recommendations tailored to individual needs.

Chapter 6

Kidney Health and Lifestyle

The phrase "kidney health and lifestyle" refers to the connection between your dietary preferences and behavioral patterns and the condition of your kidneys. Filtering waste materials and extra fluid from the blood, controlling blood pressure, balancing electrolytes, and generating hormones that promote red blood cell synthesis are all important functions of the kidneys. The maintenance of healthy kidneys is crucial for overall well-being.

Stress Management Techniques: Reducing Stress for Better Kidney Health

Chronic stress can have a significant impact on kidney health, as it can lead to elevated blood pressure, compromised immune function, and hormonal imbalances. Therefore, implementing effective stress management techniques is essential for promoting better kidney health and overall well-being.

Here are some strategies to reduce stress:

1. **Exercise:** Engaging in regular physical activity helps reduce stress by releasing endorphins, which are natural mood-enhancing chemicals in the brain. Exercise can also improve sleep quality and boost overall resilience to stress. Aim for at least 30 minutes of moderate-intensity exercise, such as walking, swimming, or cycling, on most days of the week.

2. **Relaxation Techniques:** Practicing relaxation techniques can help calm the mind and reduce stress levels. Deep breathing exercises, meditation, yoga, and progressive muscle relaxation are effective techniques that can be incorporated into daily routines. These practices promote relaxation, reduce muscle tension, and improve mental clarity.

3. **Time Management:** Feeling overwhelmed by a busy schedule can contribute to stress. Implementing effective time management strategies, such as prioritizing tasks, setting realistic goals, and delegating responsibilities, can help create a sense of control and reduce stress levels.

4. **Social Support:** Sharing your feelings and experiences with trusted friends, family members, or support groups can provide emotional support and alleviate stress. Surround yourself with positive and understanding individuals who can offer encouragement and help you navigate challenging situations.

5. **Healthy Lifestyle Habits:** Maintaining a healthy lifestyle can significantly reduce stress levels. Ensure you prioritize adequate sleep, follow a balanced diet rich in fruits, vegetables, whole grains, and lean proteins, and limit the consumption of caffeine, alcohol, and tobacco. These habits support overall well-being and resilience to stress.

6. **Hobbies and Recreation:** Engaging in activities that bring joy and relaxation can help distract from stressors and promote a sense of fulfillment. Find time for hobbies, such as reading, painting, gardening, or listening to music, to create a healthy balance in your life and reduce stress.

7. **Seek Professional Help:** If stress becomes overwhelming and affects your daily life, consider seeking professional help. A mental health professional can provide guidance, support, and techniques tailored to your specific needs.

Remember, managing stress is a continuous process, and what works for one person may not work for another. Explore different techniques, be patient with yourself, and be proactive in finding what brings you peace and relaxation. By prioritizing stress management, you can protect your kidney health and improve your overall quality of life.

Adequate sleep and rest: the impact of sleep on overall well-being

Sleep is a fundamental pillar of our overall well-being and plays a vital role in maintaining good physical and mental health. It is during sleep that our bodies undergo essential processes of repair, restoration, and consolidation of memories. Insufficient or poor-quality sleep can have a significant impact on various aspects of our lives.

Below are some key points highlighting the importance of adequate sleep and rest:

1. **Physical Health:** Sleep is crucial for the proper functioning of our immune system, as it helps strengthen our body's defenses against illnesses and infections. Sufficient sleep supports the healing and repair of tissues, aids in hormone regulation, and contributes to maintaining a healthy weight. Chronic sleep deprivation has been linked to an increased risk of developing conditions such as obesity, diabetes, cardiovascular diseases, and even certain cancers.

2. **Mental and Emotional Well-being:** Sleep plays a crucial role in cognitive function, memory consolidation, and emotional regulation. Sufficient sleep enhances our ability to concentrate, make decisions, and solve problems effectively. It also promotes emotional stability and resilience, while inadequate sleep can lead to mood swings, irritability, anxiety, and even depression. Quality sleep is essential for maintaining optimal mental health and overall emotional well-being.

3. **Energy and Productivity:** A good night's sleep is closely tied to our energy levels and overall productivity. When we are well-rested, we experience higher levels of alertness,

focus, and creativity, enabling us to perform better in our daily activities, whether at work, school, or personal endeavors. On the other hand, sleep deprivation can lead to decreased productivity, impaired cognitive function, and an increased risk of accidents and errors.

4. **Stress Reduction:** Sufficient sleep plays a crucial role in managing stress. When we sleep, our bodies undergo physiological processes that help regulate stress hormones and promote relaxation. Conversely, inadequate sleep can disrupt this balance, leading to increased stress levels, heightened emotional reactivity, and a reduced ability to cope with everyday challenges. Prioritizing quality sleep can significantly contribute to stress reduction and improve our ability to handle stressful situations effectively.

5. **Overall Quality of Life:** Getting enough sleep is essential for maintaining an overall high quality of life. It positively impacts our physical health, mental well-being, relationships, and daily functioning. Adequate sleep allows us to wake up feeling refreshed, rejuvenated, and ready to tackle the day ahead, leading to a more fulfilling and rewarding life experience.

Adequate sleep and rest are not only essential for our overall well-being but also have a significant impact on kidney health. The kidneys play a crucial role in maintaining fluid balance, regulating blood pressure, and filtering waste products from the blood.

Here's how sleep affects the well-being of the kidneys:

1. **Blood Pressure** Regulation: During sleep, our bodies naturally lower blood pressure levels. Consistently getting sufficient sleep allows the kidneys to effectively regulate blood pressure, reducing the risk of hypertension. Chronic sleep deprivation can disrupt this process and contribute to high blood pressure, which puts strain on the kidneys over time.

2. **Fluid Balance:** Adequate sleep supports proper fluid balance in the body. The kidneys help maintain this balance by filtering excess fluid through urine. Insufficient sleep can disrupt this process, leading to fluid retention and potential strain on the kidneys. It is crucial to maintain healthy fluid balance by getting enough sleep, which allows the kidneys to function optimally.

3. **Hormonal Regulation:** Sleep plays a role in hormonal regulation, and this includes hormones that impact kidney function. Adequate sleep supports the balance of hormones like aldosterone, which helps regulate sodium and potassium levels in the body. Imbalances in these hormones due to inadequate sleep can affect kidney function and contribute to electrolyte imbalances.

4. **Inflammation and Oxidative Stress:** Lack of sleep can contribute to increased inflammation and oxidative stress throughout the body, including the kidneys. These factors can have a negative impact on kidney health and increase

the risk of developing kidney disease or exacerbating existing kidney conditions.

5. **Kidney Disease Progression:** Insufficient sleep has been associated with the progression of kidney disease. Chronic kidney disease (CKD) is a condition in which the kidneys gradually lose their ability to function properly. Poor sleep quality and duration have been linked to a higher risk of CKD progression. Prioritizing adequate sleep can help slow down the progression of kidney disease and support overall kidney health.

It is important to note that individuals with pre-existing kidney conditions should consult with their healthcare professionals for personalized advice and recommendations regarding sleep and kidney health.

To promote better sleep and support kidney health, establish a regular sleep routine, create a sleep-friendly environment, and prioritize sufficient sleep duration (typically 7-9 hours for adults). Practice good sleep hygiene, such as avoiding stimulants close to bedtime and engaging in relaxation techniques before sleep. Ensure your sleep environment is comfortable, quiet, and conducive to restful sleep.

By prioritizing adequate sleep, you can contribute to the overall well-being of your kidneys and reduce the risk of kidney-related complications

Balancing Work and Personal Life: Finding Harmony for Better Health Outcomes

Finding a balance between work and personal life is crucial for maintaining good health and well-being. In today's fast-paced and demanding world, many individuals experience high levels of stress, burnout, and negative health outcomes due to an imbalance between their professional and personal commitments.

Below are some key points highlighting the importance of balancing work and personal life for better health outcomes:

1. **Stress Reduction:** Chronic work-related stress can have detrimental effects on physical and mental health. Finding a healthy balance allows for adequate rest, relaxation, and stress reduction, which can help prevent the onset of stress-related health conditions. By prioritizing personal time and self-care, individuals can better manage stress and promote overall well-being.

2. **Mental Health:** Balancing work and personal life is essential for maintaining good mental health. Constantly prioritizing work over personal needs can lead to feelings of overwhelm, anxiety, and burnout. Taking time for leisure activities, hobbies, spending quality time with loved ones, and engaging in self-care practices can improve mental well-being, enhance resilience, and prevent mental health issues.

3. **Physical Health:** Neglecting personal health due to work demands can have serious consequences for physical well-being. Finding a balance allows individuals to prioritize regular exercise, healthy eating habits, and sufficient sleep—all of which are crucial for maintaining optimal physical health. By taking care of their bodies, individuals can reduce the risk of developing chronic diseases and improve overall health outcomes.

4. **Relationship Building:** Balancing work and personal life enables individuals to nurture meaningful relationships with family, friends, and loved ones. Strong social connections provide support, emotional well-being, and a sense of belonging, which are all essential for better health outcomes. Investing time and energy into relationships can bring joy, improve overall life satisfaction, and provide a support system during challenging times.

5. **Productivity and Performance:** Achieving a balance between work and personal life can actually enhance productivity and performance in the long run. When individuals prioritize their personal needs and engage in activities that bring them joy and fulfillment, they return to work with increased focus, creativity, and motivation. Taking regular breaks and allowing time for self-rejuvenation can prevent burnout, boost job satisfaction, and lead to better professional outcomes.

6. **Boundaries and Time Management:** Establishing clear boundaries between work and personal life is essential for

achieving balance. Setting realistic goals, prioritizing tasks, and effectively managing time can help individuals allocate sufficient time for work responsibilities and personal activities. By creating a structured schedule and adhering to it, individuals can maintain a sense of control and prevent work from encroaching on personal time.

Finding a balance between work and personal life is a continuous process that requires self-awareness, prioritization, and effective time management. It may involve setting boundaries, practicing self-care, and seeking support when needed. Ultimately, achieving harmony between work and personal life contributes to better health outcomes, increased overall well-being, and a more fulfilling and satisfying life.

Poor Dieting

A poor diet can have detrimental effects on kidney health. Here are some specific ways in which a poor diet can impact the kidneys:

1. **High Sodium Intake:** Consuming excessive amounts of sodium (commonly found in processed and packaged foods) can increase blood pressure and put strain on the kidneys. This can lead to kidney damage and increase the risk of kidney disease.

2. **Processed Foods:** Processed foods often contain high levels of unhealthy fats, sodium, and additives. Regular consumption of these foods can contribute to

inflammation, obesity, diabetes, and high blood pressure, all of which are risk factors for kidney disease.

3. **Saturated Fats:** Diets high in saturated fats, commonly found in fatty meats, full-fat dairy products, and fried foods, can increase cholesterol levels and contribute to the development of cardiovascular disease. Since the kidneys rely on healthy blood vessels for proper functioning, a diet high in saturated fats can impair kidney health.

4. **Excessive Protein Consumption:** While protein is essential for the body, consuming excessive amounts of protein, especially from animal sources, can strain the kidneys. High protein intake can increase the workload on the kidneys and may accelerate the progression of kidney disease in individuals who already have compromised kidney function.

5. **Lack of Fruits, Vegetables, and Whole Grains:** Fruits, vegetables, and whole grains are rich in vitamins, minerals, fiber, and antioxidants, which support overall health, including kidney health. Their absence in the diet can deprive the body of essential nutrients and contribute to the development of chronic conditions such as obesity, diabetes, and high blood pressure, all of which can harm the kidneys.

By adopting a balanced diet that includes moderate amounts of sodium, limited processed foods, healthy fats, and a variety of fruits, vegetables, whole grains, and lean proteins, you can help protect your kidneys and reduce the risk of kidney damage. It's always advisable to consult with a healthcare professional or a registered dietitian for personalized dietary recommendations based on your specific health needs and goals.

Smoking

Smoking is detrimental to kidney health. Here's how smoking can impact the kidneys:

1. **Reduced Blood Flow:** Smoking damages blood vessels and reduces blood flow to various organs, including the kidneys. Decreased blood flow hampers the kidneys' ability to effectively filter waste products and maintain proper kidney function. Over time, this can contribute to kidney damage and impair their ability to perform vital functions.

2. **Accelerated Kidney Disease Progression:** Smoking has been linked to an increased risk of kidney disease and can hasten the progression of existing kidney conditions. It can worsen conditions like chronic kidney disease (CKD) and increase the likelihood of developing end-stage renal disease (ESRD), which may require dialysis or kidney transplantation.

3. **Increased Risk of Kidney Cancer:** Smoking is a significant risk factor for kidney cancer. The harmful chemicals present in tobacco smoke can damage DNA and lead to the formation of cancerous cells in the kidneys.

Quitting smoking can help reduce the risk of developing kidney cancer.

4. **Elevated Blood Pressure:** Smoking can elevate blood pressure, which is a major risk factor for kidney disease. High blood pressure can damage the blood vessels in the kidneys and impair their ability to function properly.

Quitting smoking is crucial for improving kidney health and reducing the risk of complications. When you quit smoking, the risk of kidney damage decreases over time, and blood flow to the kidneys improves. It's never too late to quit smoking, and the benefits for kidney health and overall well-being are significant.

If you're a smoker and looking to quit, consider seeking support from healthcare professionals, joining smoking cessation programs, or using medications or nicotine replacement therapies. They can provide guidance, resources, and strategies to help you quit smoking successfully and improve your kidney health.

Excessive Alcohol Consumption

Excessive alcohol consumption can have negative effects on kidney health. Here's how alcohol can impact the kidneys:

1. **High Blood Pressure:** Drinking alcohol in excess can elevate blood pressure, which is a significant risk factor for kidney disease. High blood pressure can damage the blood vessels in the kidneys and impair their ability to function properly.

2. **Liver Disease:** Alcohol abuse can lead to liver damage or liver disease, such as alcoholic hepatitis or cirrhosis. Liver dysfunction can indirectly affect kidney function as the liver and kidneys work together to filter and eliminate waste products from the body.

3. **Dehydration:** Alcohol is a diuretic, meaning it increases urine production and can lead to dehydration. Dehydration can cause concentrated urine, impair kidney function, and increase the risk of kidney stones and urinary tract infections.

4. **Interference with Medications:** Excessive alcohol consumption can interfere with the effectiveness of certain medications, including those prescribed for kidney-related conditions. It's important to follow healthcare professionals' recommendations regarding alcohol consumption while taking medications.

To promote kidney health, it's important to limit alcohol intake and practice moderation. The Centers for Disease Control and Prevention (CDC) defines moderate drinking as up to one drink per day for women and up to two drinks per day for men. It's essential to be aware of the standard drink sizes and stay within these limits to protect your kidneys and overall health.

If you're struggling with alcohol abuse or finding it difficult to moderate your alcohol consumption, seeking support from healthcare professionals, support groups, or specialized alcohol addiction programs can be beneficial. They can provide guidance, resources, and assistance in addressing alcohol-related concerns and improving kidney health.

Abuse or Overuse of Medications and Supplements

Overuse or improper use of medications and supplements can have adverse effects on kidney health. Here's how it can impact the kidneys:

1. Nonsteroidal Anti-Inflammatory Drugs (NSAIDs): NSAIDs, such as ibuprofen and naproxen, are commonly used to relieve pain and reduce inflammation. However, prolonged or excessive use of NSAIDs can cause kidney damage, especially in individuals with pre-existing kidney conditions or those who are dehydrated. It's important to follow the recommended dosage and duration provided by healthcare professionals and avoid long-term or high-dose use of NSAIDs without medical supervision.

2. **Certain Antibiotics:** Some antibiotics, when used inappropriately or for extended periods, can cause kidney damage. Examples include aminoglycosides and vancomycin. It's crucial to follow the prescribed dosage and duration of antibiotics and consult a healthcare professional if you have concerns or experience any adverse effects.

3. **Contrast Dyes:** Certain imaging procedures, such as computed tomography (CT) scans, may require the use of contrast dyes. These dyes can cause kidney damage, particularly in individuals with pre-existing kidney

conditions or those who are dehydrated. It's important to inform healthcare providers about any kidney issues before undergoing such procedures.

4. **Herbal Supplements:** Some herbal supplements can have adverse effects on kidney health, especially when taken in excessive amounts or combined with certain medications. Examples include high doses of creatine, certain Chinese herbal remedies, and some weight loss supplements. It's important to consult with a healthcare professional before taking any herbal supplements, especially if you have kidney disease or are at risk of developing it.

To protect kidney health, it's essential to use medications and supplements as directed by healthcare professionals. Here are some recommendations:

- Follow a prescribed dosage and duration for medications.
- Inform healthcare providers about any kidney conditions or concerns.
- Avoid self-medication and consult a healthcare professional before taking new medications or supplements.
- Stay well-hydrated, especially when taking medications known to impact kidney function.
- Be cautious with over-the-counter pain relievers and consult a healthcare professional if you need prolonged or frequent use.

By practicing responsible medication and supplement use, you can help safeguard kidney health and minimize the risk of kidney damage.

Lifestyle towards Hydration

Some people find it difficult or uncomfortable to drink water, let alone to drink enough of it. The body is negatively impacted by this in many ways, but the kidneys are particularly affected since it interferes with their natural operation.

Below are ways inadequate hydration can impact health of the kidneys significantly:

1. **Concentrated Urine:** When the body is dehydrated, the kidneys conserve water by producing concentrated urine. Concentrated urine contains higher levels of waste products and minerals, which can contribute to the formation of kidney stones. These stones can cause pain, blockage, and potentially damage the kidneys.

2. **Impaired Waste Removal:** Adequate hydration is essential for the kidneys to effectively filter waste products and toxins from the bloodstream. When the body is dehydrated, the kidneys may struggle to remove waste efficiently, leading to a buildup of harmful substances in the body.

3. **Increased Risk of Urinary Tract Infections (UTIs):** Dehydration can reduce urine production and decrease the flushing action that helps remove bacteria from the urinary

tract. This can increase the risk of UTIs, which can potentially affect the kidneys if left untreated.

To maintain proper kidney function and reduce the risk of complications, it is crucial to drink enough water throughout the day. The adequate amount of fluid intake varies depending on individual factors such as age, activity level, climate, and overall health. As a general guideline, aim to consume about 8 cups (64 ounces) of water per day, or follow your healthcare provider's recommendations.

It's important to note that individual fluid requirements may vary. Factors such as certain medical conditions, medications, and lifestyle factors can influence the amount of water you need. Consult with your healthcare provider to determine the appropriate fluid intake for your specific situation.

In addition to water, you can also obtain hydration from other sources such as herbal teas, fruits, vegetables, and soups. However, be mindful of consuming excessive amounts of caffeinated beverages and sugary drinks, as they can have diuretic effects and contribute to dehydration.

Remember to listen to your body's thirst signals and make it a habit to drink water regularly throughout the day. Adequate hydration is essential for maintaining proper kidney function and overall well-being.

Lack of Physical Activity

A sedentary lifestyle can have significant consequences for kidney health. Here's how lack of physical activity and leading a sedentary lifestyle can impact the kidneys:

1. **Obesity:** Lack of regular physical activity is a contributing factor to weight gain and obesity. Obesity is a known risk factor for kidney disease. Excess body weight puts strain on the kidneys and increases the likelihood of developing conditions like diabetes and high blood pressure, which further increase the risk of kidney damage.

2. **Diabetes:** A sedentary lifestyle is associated with an increased risk of developing type 2 diabetes. Diabetes is a leading cause of kidney disease. Regular exercise can help improve insulin sensitivity, maintain healthy blood sugar levels, and reduce the risk of diabetes-related kidney damage.

3. **High Blood Pressure:** Lack of physical activity contributes to the development of high blood pressure (hypertension), which is a major risk factor for kidney disease. Regular exercise helps control blood pressure levels, improve cardiovascular health, and reduce the strain on the kidneys.

4. **Impaired Blood Circulation:** A sedentary lifestyle can lead to poor circulation and reduced blood flow to the kidneys. Adequate blood flow is crucial for optimal kidney function. Regular exercise promotes healthy blood

circulation, ensuring that the kidneys receive sufficient oxygen and nutrients for proper functioning.

5. **Inflammation and Oxidative Stress:** Sedentary behavior has been associated with increased inflammation and oxidative stress in the body, which can contribute to kidney damage over time. Regular exercise helps reduce inflammation, promote antioxidant defenses, and support kidney health.

Incorporating regular physical activity into your lifestyle is essential for maintaining kidney health and overall well-being. Aim for at least 150 minutes of moderate-intensity aerobic exercise or 75 minutes of vigorous-intensity aerobic exercise per week, along with muscle-strengthening activities on two or more days.

Find activities you enjoy, such as walking, jogging, swimming, cycling, dancing, or participating in sports, and make them a regular part of your routine. Even simple lifestyle changes like taking regular breaks from sitting and incorporating more movement throughout the day can have a positive impact on kidney health.

If you have any underlying health conditions or concerns, it is advisable to consult with a healthcare professional to determine the appropriate exercise plan for your specific needs. Regular physical activity, along with a balanced diet, can help maintain a healthy weight, promote cardiovascular health, and support optimal kidney function.

Delaying or Ignoring Medical Conditions

Absolutely, delaying or ignoring medical conditions can have a significant impact on kidney health. Here's how the delay or neglect of chronic conditions can affect the kidneys:

1. **Diabetes:** Untreated or poorly managed diabetes can lead to diabetic nephropathy, a condition that damages the kidneys. High blood sugar levels over time can impair the small blood vessels in the kidneys, affecting their ability to filter waste from the blood. Timely management of diabetes through proper medication, blood sugar control, and lifestyle changes is essential to prevent or slow down the progression of kidney damage.

2. **Hypertension (High Blood Pressure):** Uncontrolled high blood pressure can damage the blood vessels in the kidneys, leading to kidney disease. The kidneys play a vital role in regulating blood pressure, and when blood pressure is consistently elevated, it can strain the kidneys and impair their function. Managing blood pressure through lifestyle modifications and medications, as prescribed by a healthcare professional, is crucial for preserving kidney health.

3. **Urinary Tract Infections (UTIs):** Ignoring or delaying treatment for urinary tract infections can lead to complications that can affect the kidneys. UTIs can travel up the urinary tract and potentially cause kidney infections,

which can be more serious and may result in kidney damage. Prompt identification and treatment of UTIs can help prevent such complications.

4. **Kidney Stones:** Neglecting the symptoms of kidney stones and delaying medical attention can lead to complications and potential kidney damage. Kidney stones can block the urinary tract and cause severe pain, infections, and damage to the kidneys. Timely intervention by a healthcare professional can help manage and prevent complications associated with kidney stones.

Regular check-ups and timely treatment of medical conditions are crucial for preserving kidney health. It's important to follow up with healthcare professionals, adhere to prescribed treatments, and maintain regular monitoring of blood sugar levels, blood pressure, and kidney function through urine and blood tests. These measures help detect and manage any potential kidney issues early, improving the chances of preserving kidney function and overall health.

If you have chronic conditions or any concerns about your kidney health, it's advisable to consult with a healthcare professional who can provide appropriate guidance, personalized treatment plans, and regular monitoring to ensure the best possible kidney care.

Timely Medical Help

Failure to seek timely medical help for kidney-related symptoms can have serious consequences. Here's why it's important to promptly address symptoms that may indicate kidney issues:

1. **Early Detection of Kidney Disease:** Many kidney diseases are silent and do not cause noticeable symptoms in the early stages. By paying attention to warning signs, such as persistent urinary problems, changes in urine color, or pain in the kidney area, you can catch potential kidney issues early on. Early detection allows for timely intervention, management, and the potential to slow down the progression of kidney disease.

2. **Prompt Treatment and Management:** Seeking medical attention for kidney-related symptoms allows healthcare professionals to accurately diagnose the underlying cause and recommend appropriate treatment options. Prompt treatment can help alleviate symptoms, prevent complications, and manage the condition effectively.

3. **Prevention of Further Damage:** Delayed diagnosis and treatment can lead to the progression of kidney disease, potentially causing irreversible damage to the kidneys. By seeking timely medical help, you increase the chances of preventing further deterioration of kidney function and minimizing the risk of complications.

4. **Management of Symptoms:** Kidney-related symptoms, such as pain or discomfort in the kidney area or swelling in the hands and feet, can significantly impact quality of life.

Prompt medical attention enables healthcare professionals to address the symptoms and provide appropriate interventions to manage discomfort and improve well-being.

If you experience persistent urinary problems, changes in urine color, pain or discomfort in the kidney area, swelling in the hands and feet, or any other concerning symptoms related to the kidneys, it's important to consult with a healthcare professional. They can conduct the necessary evaluations, order relevant tests, and provide appropriate guidance and treatment options based on your specific situation.

Remember, early detection and timely medical intervention are key to managing kidney issues effectively and preserving kidney health. Do not hesitate to seek medical help if you have any concerns or symptoms related to your kidneys.

Chapter 7

When to Seek Medical Help

Maintaining your health and wellbeing depends on your ability to see issues and determine when to seek medical advice. You can use the following general principles to determine probable issues and when it's best to consult a doctor:

1. **Worsening or persistent symptoms:** If you are experiencing symptoms that are getting worse or have not improved over time, it may indicate a more serious underlying issue. For example, if you have a respiratory infection and your cough and difficulty breathing are getting worse, it's time to consult a healthcare professional.

2. **Severe pain or discomfort:** If you are experiencing severe or persistent pain that is not alleviated by over-the-counter medications, it may be a sign of a more significant problem and requires medical attention.

3. **Fever:** A fever can be a sign of an infection, and if it is high-grade or persistent, it's important to seek medical advice, especially if accompanied by other symptoms.

4. **Difficulty in breathing:** Shortness of breath, wheezing, or difficulty breathing could be indicative of various

respiratory or cardiovascular issues. Seek immediate medical attention if you experience these symptoms.

5. **Chest pain:** Chest pain can be a sign of a heart attack or other serious cardiac issues. If you have chest pain, especially if it radiates to your arm, neck, jaw, or back, call emergency services immediately.

6. **Sudden or severe headaches:** If you experience a sudden, severe headache, especially if it's accompanied by other symptoms like vision changes, difficulty speaking, or confusion, seek medical attention promptly as it could be a sign of a stroke or other neurological issues.

7. **Uncontrolled bleeding:** If you have a wound or injury that is bleeding excessively and does not stop with pressure, you should seek immediate medical care.

8. **Changes in bowel or bladder habits:** If you notice significant changes in your bowel movements or urination patterns, especially if there is blood in the stool or urine, it may indicate a gastrointestinal or urological problem.

9. **Persistent fatigue or weakness:** If you are experiencing unexplained and persistent fatigue or weakness, it could be a sign of an underlying medical condition that requires evaluation.

10. **Unexplained weight loss:** If you are losing weight without trying or without changes in diet or exercise, it could be a cause for concern and should be evaluated by a healthcare professional.

11. **Skin changes:** New or unusual skin growths, changes in moles, or skin discolorations should be checked by a dermatologist, as they may indicate skin cancer or other skin disorders.
12. **Mental health concerns:** If you or someone you know is experiencing significant changes in mood, prolonged sadness, anxiety, or thoughts of self-harm, seeking mental health support is crucial.

Remember that this list is not exhaustive, and if you have any concerns about your health or well-being, it's always better to err on the side of caution and consult a healthcare professional. Your health is precious, and early detection and treatment of potential complications can lead to better outcomes.

The importance of regular check-ups and kidney function tests

Regular check-ups and kidney function tests are of utmost importance for maintaining overall health and detecting kidney-related issues at an early stage. The kidneys play a crucial role in filtering waste products and excess fluids from the blood, regulating blood pressure, producing hormones, and maintaining electrolyte balance in the body. Kidney function tests are designed to assess how well the kidneys are performing their functions.

Some key reasons why regular check-ups and kidney function tests are important are as follows:

1. **Early detection of kidney problems:** Kidney diseases often progress silently and may not exhibit noticeable symptoms in the early stages. Regular kidney function tests can detect abnormalities in kidney function before significant damage occurs, allowing for early intervention and better management of the condition.

2. **Prevention of kidney disease** progression: If kidney problems are detected early, lifestyle changes, medications, and other treatments can be initiated to slow down or prevent further kidney damage. This can help avoid complications such as kidney failure, which may require dialysis or transplantation.

3. **Monitoring chronic conditions:** Individuals with conditions like diabetes, hypertension (high blood pressure), and heart disease are at higher risk of developing kidney problems. Regular kidney function tests are essential for monitoring kidney health in these patients and adapting treatment plans accordingly.

4. **Medication management:** Some medications, including certain pain relievers and antibiotics, can be harmful to the kidneys. Regular check-ups and kidney function tests help healthcare providers monitor how medications are affecting kidney function and adjust dosages if necessary.

5. **Assessing overall health:** Kidney function tests are often included in routine health check-ups, along with other tests like blood pressure measurements, blood glucose tests, and cholesterol checks.

6. These comprehensive assessments provide a clearer picture of an individual's overall health status.

7. **Evaluation of kidney health before surgery:** Before undergoing surgery, especially major procedures that may put additional stress on the kidneys, it is essential to assess kidney function to ensure they can handle the stress of anesthesia and potential fluid imbalances during the operation.

8. **Tracking changes over time:** Regular kidney function tests allow healthcare providers to monitor kidney health over time. This helps in identifying any trends or changes that might require further investigation or intervention.

In summary, regular check-ups and kidney function tests are critical for maintaining kidney health, detecting kidney-related problems early, and taking appropriate measures to prevent or slow down the progression of kidney diseases. They also contribute to overall health and well-being by providing valuable insights into the body's functioning and identifying potential health risks before they become serious issues. If you have concerns about your kidney health or are at higher risk of kidney problems, talk to your healthcare provider about the appropriate screening and monitoring schedule for you.

Treatment options for kidney infections: medical interventions and antibiotics.

Kidney infections, also known as pyelonephritis, are serious bacterial infections that affect the kidneys. They require prompt medical attention and treatment to prevent complications and further kidney damage. The primary treatment options for kidney infections include medical interventions and antibiotics. Here's an overview of the typical treatment approach:

1. **Antibiotics:** Antibiotics are the mainstay of treatment for kidney infections. The choice of antibiotic will depend on the severity of the infection, the suspected bacteria causing the infection, and any known drug allergies.

Commonly prescribed antibiotics for kidney infections include:

- Fluoroquinolones (e.g., ciprofloxacin, levofloxacin)
- Trimethoprim-sulfamethoxazole (TMP-SMX)
- Cephalosporins (e.g., ceftriaxone, cefalexin)
- Beta-lactam antibiotics (e.g., amoxicillin, ampicillin)

It's essential to complete the full course of antibiotics as prescribed by the healthcare provider, even if you start feeling better before finishing the medication. This helps ensure that the infection is completely eradicated and reduces the risk of recurrence or antibiotic resistance.

2. **Hospitalization:** In severe cases of kidney infection or if the patient has other health complications, hospitalization may be necessary. Hospital treatment provides closer monitoring, intravenous (IV) administration of antibiotics for more potent and rapid delivery, and supportive care to manage dehydration, fever, and pain.

3. **Pain management:** Kidney infections can be painful, and pain management is an essential part of the treatment. Over-the-counter pain relievers like acetaminophen or ibuprofen may be used to alleviate discomfort. However, it's crucial to avoid non-steroidal anti-inflammatory drugs (NSAIDs) if kidney function is impaired, as they can further harm the kidneys.

4. **Fluids and hydration:** Staying well-hydrated is vital during kidney infection treatment. Adequate fluid intake helps flush out bacteria and toxins from the urinary system and supports kidney function. If necessary, intravenous fluids may be administered in the hospital setting to maintain hydration.

5. **Follow-up care:** After completing the course of antibiotics, it's essential to have a follow-up appointment with the healthcare provider. Follow-up tests, such as urine analysis and cultures, may be conducted to ensure the infection has resolved and to monitor kidney function.

It's crucial to seek medical attention promptly if you suspect a kidney infection, as untreated infections can lead to severe complications, such as kidney damage, sepsis (blood infection), or abscess formation. Never self-diagnose or self-treat a kidney infection, as improper management can lead to serious consequences.

Always consult a healthcare professional for an accurate diagnosis and appropriate treatment plan based on your specific condition and medical history.

Conclusion

Empowering individuals to take proactive steps in preventing kidney infections and emphasizing the significance of kidney health for overall wellness are essential components of promoting a healthier society. By encouraging the adoption of healthy habits and lifestyle choices, we can support optimal kidney function and reduce the risk of kidney-related complications.

Taking responsibility for our own health and well-being is a powerful step towards preventing kidney infections. Practicing good hygiene, staying hydrated, and practicing safe sex are simple yet effective measures that can make a significant difference. Additionally, being mindful of our diet and managing chronic conditions like diabetes and high blood pressure are crucial in safeguarding kidney health.

Recognizing the vital role kidneys play in maintaining the body's internal balance, we must prioritize kidney health as an integral part of our overall well-being. Healthy kidneys not only help remove waste and toxins but also regulate blood pressure, electrolyte balance, and red blood cell production, contributing to our energy levels and overall vitality.

By fostering a culture of health consciousness and regular medical check-ups, we can proactively identify any kidney-related issues and intervene early, preventing the progression of kidney diseases.

Let us all commit to making informed choices and adopting healthier lifestyles to protect our kidneys and promote overall wellness. Together, we can build a healthier future and ensure that kidney health remains at the forefront of our collective efforts to lead fulfilling and vibrant lives.

Note: The content provided is for informational purposes only and should not be considered as medical advice. It is always recommended to consult with a healthcare professional for personalized guidance and treatment options.

References

https://drmirdamadi.com/medicine/renal-system/

https://www.drsaurindalal.com/kidney-transplant.html

https://www.health.com/kidney-infection-overview-7498691

https://www.medicalnewstoday.com/articles/305488#location

https://www.medicalnewstoday.com/articles/305488#structure

https://www.nhsinform.scot/illnesses-and-conditions/kidneys-bladder-and-prostate/kidney-infection

https://www.niddk.nih.gov/health-information/kidney-disease/kidneys-how-they-work

https://www.verywellhealth.com/what-is-the-structure-and-function-of-the-kidneys-2085832